The Rockingham mausoleum, Wentworth, South Yorkshire, was built by John Carr in 1785–91. Inside are a statue of the second Marquis of Rockingham (1730–82), Prime Minister in 1765–6 and again in 1782, and busts of his friends. The mausoleum, which still retains its atmospheric gloom even after restoration in 1989, is now in the care of the Wentworth Monuments Society.

Mausoleums

Lynn F. Pearson

A Shire book

Contents

Mausoleums – a history 3

A gazetteer of mausoleums in Great Britain 10

England 10

Scotland 34

Wales 39

Further reading 40

British Library Cataloguing in Publication Data: Pearson, Lynn F. Mausoleums. – (A Shire book; 396) 1. Mausoleums – Great Britain – History 2. Mausoleums – Great Britain – Guidebooks I. Title 726.8'0941. ISBN 0 7478 0518 0.

Cover: *The derelict Delaval mausoleum, Seaton Delaval Hall, Northumberland, was built for Sir John Delaval in 1766. The architect is unknown but, given that the hall itself was built by Sir John Vanbrugh (1664–1726) for Admiral George Delaval in 1718–29, perhaps he discussed the eventual design of the mausoleum with the Admiral. Vanbrugh is indeed known to have originated the idea of building a mausoleum at Castle Howard, although this structure was finally designed by Hawksmoor and erected in 1729–45.*

ACKNOWLEDGEMENTS

The author would like to thank Trevor Ermel of Monochrome, the staff of the National Monuments Record (London searchroom), the Tiles and Architectural Ceramics Society, the Mausolea and Monuments Trust; Clare Graham, Dennis Hadley, Tony and Kathy Herbert, Sue Hudson, Hans van Lemmen, Biddy Macfarlane, Jim and Margaret Perry, and Jeff Sechiari. The photograph on page 28 is by Tony Herbert. The photographs on pages 3, 5 (top), 7 (bottom), 8, 10, 11 (both), 12 (both), 13 (bottom), 15, 17, 18 (both), 19, 22 (top), 23 (top), 25 (left), 26 (bottom), 30 (both), 31 (all), 32 (top), 35 and 36 (top) are by Cadbury Lamb. All other photographs, including the cover picture, are by the author. National Grid References (NGR) are included in the text to indicate the locations of some of the more remote mausoleums. They are used by permission of the Controller of Her Majesty's Stationery Office.

Published in 2002 by Shire Publications Ltd, Cromwell House, Church Street, Princes Risborough, Buckinghamshire HP27 9AA, UK. Website: www.shirebooks.co.uk
Copyright © 2002 by Lynn F. Pearson. First published 2002. Shire Album 396. ISBN 0 7478 0518 0.
Lynn F. Pearson is hereby identified as the author of this work in accordance with Section 77 of the Copyright, Designs and Patents Act 1988.

Printed in Great Britain by CIT Printing Services Ltd, Press Buildings, Merlins Bridge, Haverfordwest, Pembrokeshire SA61 1XF.

Mausoleums - a history

The first mausoleums of modern times were primitive in design, although ancient precedents for much grander buildings existed, particularly the splendid tomb erected for King Mausolos of Caria at Halicarnassos (south-west Turkey) about 353 BC, which gave its name to the mausoleum. It took the form of a huge rectangular podium, from which rose thirty-six columns capped by a pyramidal roof reaching 140 feet (43 metres) in height. A mausoleum may be defined simply as a magnificent or monumental tomb, thus allowing a broad consideration of funerary architecture, taking in smaller tombs and family chapels in churches. However, this definition seems inadequate when discussing mausoleums as a building type. A more intuitive description including elements of entrance, enclosure, mass and separation leads to the definition of a mausoleum as a substantial, discrete funerary structure containing (or intended to contain) a tomb or tombs, and which can – at least theoretically – be entered. Although this book does include many examples of mausoleums that are inside or attached to churches, the emphasis lies with those buildings that make a significant individual contribution to the landscape.

Disposal of the dead is a problem as old as humanity. The earliest inhumation (burial in the ground) in Britain took place around 24,380 BC, but evidence from this remote period suggests that cremation was more common than burial. In the Neolithic era bones were often interred within chambers beneath mounds known as long barrows (which might be classified as the first mausoleums), but they were sometimes removed and deposited with other bones, thus losing the integrity of the skeleton. Individual burials became more common in the Bronze Age, while high social status was reflected by prominent barrows and rich grave goods, a theme that runs throughout funerary history. By the time of the Roman invasion of Britain inhumation appears to have become the usual method of disposal, and distinct cemetery areas were being created; by Anglo-Saxon times, these often occupied significant positions in the landscape.

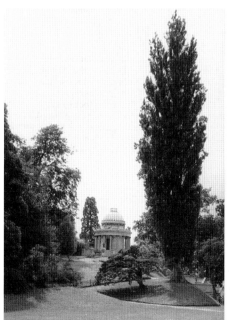

The mausoleum as garden building: the mausoleum of the Duchess of Kent, in Windsor Home Park, Berkshire, was completed in 1861. The domed, colonnaded rotunda was designed by the architect Albert Jenkins Humbert just before he began work on the nearby Royal Mausoleum for Queen Victoria, daughter of the Duchess. The interior is surprisingly bright, with red-painted walls and blue glass in the ceiling.

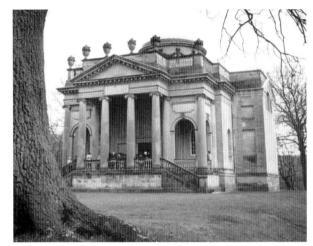

The classical chapel at Gibside, Rowlands Gill, County Durham, stands above the Bowes mausoleum. Work on the chapel, which was designed by James Paine, began in 1759 but was not completed until 1816. Access to the mausoleum is via double iron doors in the wall at the rear of the chapel.

The coming of Christianity signalled a change in approach, as the construction of a network of parish churches offered new and desirable local sites for burial. Place of burial reflected the status of the deceased: for those at the highest level, burial within religious institutions was available; for locally important families, intramural burial (within the confines of the church) was the norm; for the rest, the end was an unmarked grave in the churchyard. By the sixteenth century both churches and churchyards had become overcrowded, and intramural burials were looked on with increasing disapproval; indeed, the Church of Scotland forbade the practice in 1581. The result was the construction of an assortment of additional aisles and chapels, unroofed enclosures and eventually mausoleums in the churchyard, taking the high-status dead outside the church walls while still retaining the all-important religious connection. This was the first stage in the long-drawn-out process of retrieving death from the clutches of the Church.

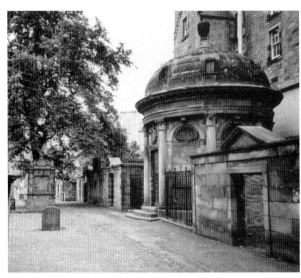

One of the earliest British mausoleums was built for Sir George Mackenzie at Greyfriars Churchyard, Edinburgh, by the designer and mason James Smith; it was completed in 1691, the year of Mackenzie's death. The domed mausoleum, which was restored in 1892, is octagonal in plan, whilst the interior is circular.

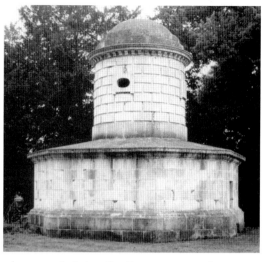

The Freeman mausoleum, Fawley, Buckinghamshire, is an early example of a freestanding churchyard mausoleum. It was built in 1750 by John Freeman (d.1752) of Fawley Court, both in memory of his father and as a family tomb; its design was based on that of an ancient Roman tomb. Freeman also redesigned the gardens of Fawley Court during the 1730s.

Some of the earliest British mausoleums are to be found in Scottish graveyards, notably Greyfriars in Edinburgh, where the domed, neo-classical Mackenzie mausoleum was completed in 1691. In England, freestanding churchyard mausoleums generally did not appear until the mid eighteenth century, an early example being the Freeman mausoleum (1750) at Fawley in Buckinghamshire. The English *had* built mausoleums before that date, not in England but in India, where – inspired by grand Mughal tombs – traders erected memorable mausoleums in a variety of styles from as early as 1659. Those at the cemetery in Surat so impressed the young John Vanbrugh, who worked in India during 1683–5, that he was able to make a sketch of them in 1711, when he was one of the Commissioners for building Fifty New Churches in the suburbs of London. Vanbrugh suggested woodland cemeteries, far from the city, where noble mausoleums could be built for the wealthy. Crucially, Vanbrugh sought to build in parkland rather than on consecrated ground.

The first such freestanding family mausoleum, a monumental structure that also functioned as a sublime object in the landscape, was erected at Castle Howard in Yorkshire. Vanbrugh

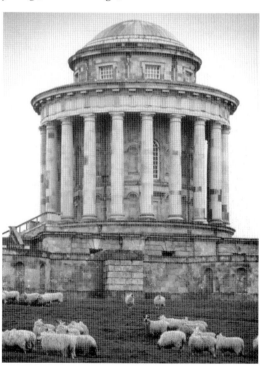

The mausoleum built in 1729–45 for the third Earl of Carlisle in the grounds of Castle Howard, North Yorkshire. The design, with twenty columns surrounding a domed, cylindrical core, was by Nicholas Hawksmoor, who died before construction was complete; the stairs and outer walls were added by Thomas Robinson and Daniel Garrett. Inside is a chapel set above the vaulted crypt, with adjoining chambers housing sixty-four niches, many empty.

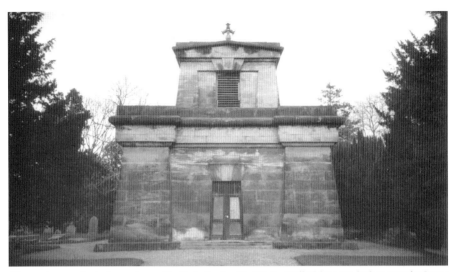

The massive neo-classical mausoleum of the Sutherlands at Trentham, Staffordshire, was built in 1808 for George Granville Leveson-Gower (1758–1833), Marquis of Stafford, later Duke of Sutherland, who inherited the Trentham estate in 1803. Its architect, Charles Heathcote Tatham, specialised in mausoleums, monuments and garden buildings, where his strict neo-classical principles could flourish.

discussed the project with the Earl of Carlisle in the early 1720s, although it was not until 1729, after Vanbrugh's death, that building began, and 1745 before it was complete. The second half of the eighteenth century then proved to be the golden age of the mausoleum, as landowners found the idea of building a mausoleum within their estate increasingly attractive, although some hedged their bets and built close to the church (and some churches were located within estates). Not only did the building act as an eye-catcher, but it provided the family with a safe haven for family remains, unsullied by contact with social inferiors.

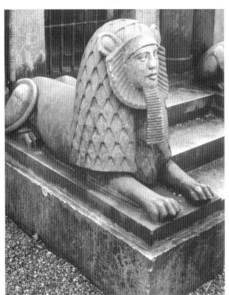

Mausoleum design became an everyday architectural activity; during 1768–1820 the Royal Academy received 164 designs for mausoleums, of which 70 were built. Architects often designed mausoleums for families on whose estates they were already erecting other buildings. The form became particularly popular in Ireland, where a series of massive mausoleums, some of unusual

A sphinx guarding the Illingworth mausoleum at Undercliffe Cemetery, Bradford, West Yorkshire. The mausoleum, which has excellent Egyptianate detailing but no inscription apart from the family name, is sited just below the main promenade.

6

The Ducrow mausoleum, Kensal Green Cemetery, London, offers a multitude of symbols: sphinx, angel, horse, beehive, torches and shells amongst them. The designer was John Cusworth, and the mausoleum was erected in 1837 by the circus owner Andrew Ducrow (1793–1842); it was originally intended for his first wife, who died in 1836.

design (probably inspired by the Mughal tombs), appeared in demesnes and graveyards. Stylistically mausoleums could be inventive, even experimental, although the neo-classical idiom was common at first, soon followed by the Greek revival style.

In the first half of the nineteenth century death became increasingly secularised. Overcrowding in churchyards and pressure from Nonconformists for unconsecrated burial grounds led to the formation of cemetery companies in the early 1820s, and the establishment of suburban garden cemeteries from the 1830s. Kensal Green Cemetery, London, opened in 1833; buyers of burial plots were allowed to erect whatever monuments they desired, and thus the aspiring middle classes – perhaps lacking social acceptance but not the wherewithal – were at last able to build fitting memorials and mausoleums. The Gothic revival of the late 1830s onward reintroduced the Gothic style to funerary architecture. Its Christian symbolism had for long been regarded as papist, but the revival harked back to an idealised medieval Christianity, and Gothic motifs became symbols of Victorian spirituality. However, the Victorian cemetery was truly diverse in style: Tudor and Greek might sit alongside Gothic and Egyptianate, which became popular for monuments because of both its direct association with pyramidal tombs and its indirect symbolic references to freemasonry.

Mausoleum building received further impetus from the two royal mausoleums at Windsor: the Duchess of Kent's was completed in 1861, while the foundations of

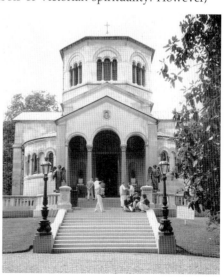

The site for the Royal Mausoleum, in the Home Park about a mile from Windsor Castle, Berkshire, was chosen by Queen Victoria soon after the death of Prince Albert in 1861. Construction took ten years and resulted in the most ornate interior of any British mausoleum. The style echoes the Italian Renaissance, with frescoes, statues, stained glass and reliefs; all is centred on the tomb chest bearing two white marble effigies of the Queen and the Prince Consort.

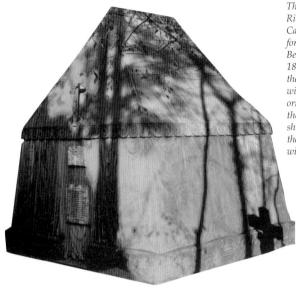

Queen Victoria's Royal Mausoleum were laid the following year. It became fashionable for the wealthy and aristocratic to use funerary monuments as a means of display as well as commemoration; during the 1860s the number of mausoleums built increased significantly, as did their size. Major architects began to work in the field, bringing stylistic flourishes such as polychromatic stonework; styles and materials were eclectic. Aside from the many varieties of stone, and sometimes brick, there were mausoleums of cast iron (although this was far more common in late-nineteenth-century America) and terracotta, while interiors became much brighter, with stained glass and mosaic work providing colour and light effects; heaven's symbolism had changed from pure classical to rich Victorian.

The most decorative British mausoleums undoubtedly date from the mid to late Victorian period, for instance the Royal Mausoleum (1862–71), the Rolle mausoleum at Bicton in Devon (a delightful Pugin work of 1850), the mausoleum of Napoleon III at Farnborough in Hampshire (1887), Sir Richard Burton's mausoleum at Mortlake in London (a heavenly Bedouin tent built around 1890), and the Monteath mausoleum near Ancrum in the Scottish Borders (1864), with its starry skylights.

The vogue for mausoleum construction began to abate in the Edwardian era, as the number of cremations increased and statements of wealth through funerary art became unfashionable. The late-nineteenth-century flood of mausoleums dried to a trickle in the early years of the twentieth century, although a few were built between the wars. The situation was different abroad, particularly in the United States, where mausoleums remained – and still remain – a popular means of commemoration; many firms now specialise in their design. Although American mausoleums tend towards extravagant, stone-built permanence, there are other options: in Mexico, graveyards house mausoleums made of colourful plastics, like glorified dolls' houses.

It is notable that no mausoleum was built following the most high-profile British death of recent times, that of Diana, Princess of Wales, in 1997. Her ashes rest in an

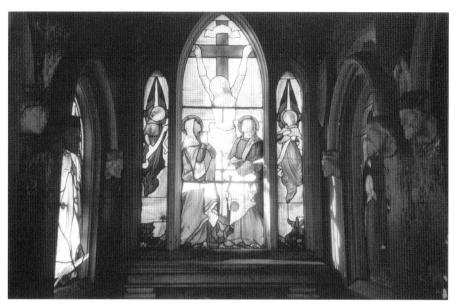

Stained glass inside the Bayona mausoleum, St Mary's Roman Catholic Cemetery, Kensal Green, London. The decorative interior also includes a brightly painted ceiling, a high-relief altar and a Minton encaustic tiled floor; it is a royal chapel in miniature.

urn near an anodyne postmodern chapel on the Althorp estate in Northamptonshire; even proposals for a memorial to the Princess became mired in controversy. It seems unlikely that modern attitudes to death and disposal will ever allow the mass creation of mausoleums in the manner of the late nineteenth century, although a few new mausoleums are currently being built on country estates, echoing eighteenth-century practice. However, even Britain is undergoing a revival of interest in burial, or more accurately alternative means of disposal; woodland cemeteries are popular and appear to be profitable. It is possible that the renewed, but now well-established, interest in gardening, garden design and garden buildings will combine with an awareness of alternative forms of burial practice to create a resurgence of enthusiasm for funerary art. We may yet be able to confront death and commemorate the dead as our ancestors did. But given modern sensibilities, maybe this process will be at arm's length, via the internet: not only do several mausoleums have their own websites, but some websites are actually mausoleums. Now you can pay to have your loved one immortalised on a plaque of your own design in a web mausoleum; perhaps these virtual memorials will escape the decay that is the inevitable fate of more substantive monuments.

A gazetteer of mausoleums in Great Britain

This gazetteer is drawn from a database of around 350 mausoleums of special architectural or historic interest. Please note that mention of a mausoleum in the gazetteer does not imply any form of public access. Many mausoleums are on private land and access may be only by prior permission (or by payment of a fee); even where grounds are open, access to a specific mausoleum may be limited. In any case, it is rare that the interior of a mausoleum is accessible. Please check before visiting to avoid disappointment.

ENGLAND
BEDFORDSHIRE
Blunham

Just south of the church of St James and St Edmund is the mausoleum built in 1805–6 by Stephen Thornton (a member of the evangelical Clapham Sect) for his father, Godfrey Thornton, a director of the Bank of England, who died in 1805. The mausoleum is a small, square, rendered structure with a hipped roof; the south elevation bears the Thornton arms. The family lived at nearby Mogerhanger Park.

Flitton

The De Grey mausoleum was built in 1614, initially for Henry Grey, fifth Earl of Kent, who died in that year; the family home was nearby Wrest Park. It is attached to the north side of the chancel of St John's Church and is in the care of English Heritage; a key to its iron gates may be ob-tained from a nearby house. Inside, the mausoleum is chilling in every sense. It contains a small art gallery of funereal monuments, including the polychromed alabaster figure of Henry Grey, reclining on a tomb chest with his wife; a pair of white marble effigies of the ninth Earl and his wife, erected 1658; and a collection of other family monuments, the latest of which dates from 1859.

Maulden

The Ailesbury (or Bruce) mausoleum on its hilltop site at St Mary's Church is an 1859 rebuilding, probably by Benjamin Ferrey, of the original mausoleum erected by Thomas Bruce, first Earl of Elgin, in 1656. This was a memorial to his second wife, Diana, and inside was a large marble monument which attempted to portray Diana, Lady Elgin, rising heavenwards. Horace Walpole found it 'ridiculous', but we cannot now judge as the

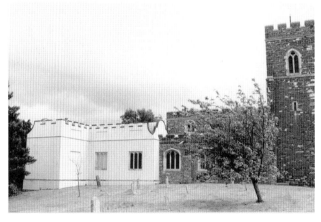

Access to the De Grey mausoleum, Flitton, Bedfordshire, is through an archway in the north side of the chancel of the adjoining church of St John the Baptist. Although both its exterior – apart from the crenellations – and interior are plain, the mausoleum contains an exceptionally fine series of funerary monuments.

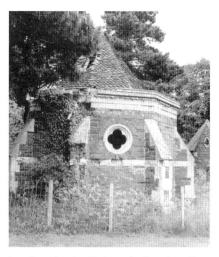

The Ailesbury mausoleum, Maulden, Bedfordshire, is an octagonal structure built of ironstone. Its link to the adjoining church was removed during its 1859 reconstruction and replaced by a south doorway; beneath the mausoleum is a crypt containing niches with the remains of many of the Bruce family.

monument has been removed (along with two other family busts), and the mausoleum has not been used since 1837. It was undergoing restoration, including the addition of replica statues, by Bedfordshire County Council during 2001.

Old Warden

The Ongley mausoleum at St Leonard's Church was built for the family in 1787; it is a small, square stone building with some classical decoration, including elegant oval windows. Within the church is an overpowering collection of Flemish and English carved woodwork from the sixteenth, seventeenth and eighteenth centuries, installed by Robert Henley, third Lord Ongley, in 1841.

Sharnbrook

The Magniac mausoleum – a massive, decorated tomb chest in the churchyard of St Peter's Church – was built in 1870. It was designed by the architect William Burges in a Sicilian version of the Romanesque style and now shelters beneath a rustic shed roof. There is also a showy 1867 monument to Hollingworth Magniac and his wife within the church.

Turvey

The magnificent nineteenth-century mausoleum of the Higgins family stands in the churchyard of All Saints' Church; all around are strangely undulating and rather intimidating yew hedges. The architectural style of the mausoleum mirrors that of local Jacobean houses. The square, mostly brick structure is topped with pinnacles and has large stone lettering on its balustrade: 'What man is he that liveth and shall not see death?'

BERKSHIRE
Wargrave

The mausoleum of the Hannen family was built by Sir Edwin Lutyens in 1906–7 and stands close to St Mary's Church.

Windsor

West of Frogmore House, in Windsor Home Park, are two mausoleums: the Royal Mausoleum and the mausoleum of the

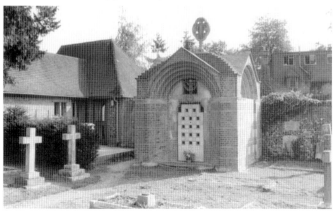

The Hannen mausoleum, Wargrave, Berkshire, was designed by Sir Edwin Lutyens in 1906–7. This elegant little building was built in brick and red tiles, its square plan and stepped doorcase giving a foretaste of Lutyens's later and much larger war memorials. Its exterior is decorated with carved stone peacocks, while entry to the domed interior is via an iron door.

11

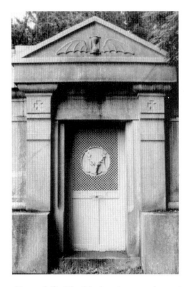
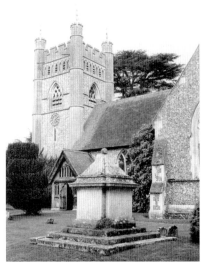

Above left: The Mackenzie mausoleum, in the churchyard at Fawley, Buckinghamshire, was built in 1862. Constructed of Aberdeen granite in vaguely Greek style, its decoration includes a sinister bat-winged hourglass. The Mackenzies' home was Fawley Court, which they extended in 1884; in addition, they helped to rebuild the church, as did the Freemans, previous residents of the house, whose mausoleum also stands in the churchyard.

Above right: The Lane family mausoleum at St Mary's Church, Hambleden, Buckinghamshire, dates from the mid eighteenth century. It is one of two mausoleums in the churchyard, both quietly classical in design and typical of small family monuments of the time.

Duchess of Kent. Following Prince Albert's death in 1861, his body was placed in the royal vault beneath St George's Chapel, Windsor, where it remained for just over a year. The Royal Mausoleum was consecrated in 1862, and Prince Albert's body was then transferred to the new crypt; work on the mausoleum was finally completed in 1871. The architect was Albert Jenkins Humbert, who designed Sandringham House shortly afterwards. He succeeded in providing an imposing exterior, basically a domed octagon topping a Greek cross plan, but the interior, designed by the Prince Consort's favourite decorative specialist, Professor Grüner of Dresden, is rather more memorable. The body of Queen Victoria was placed in the mausoleum, beside that of her husband, on her death in 1901. The Royal Mausoleum is open to the public on the nearest Wednesday to 24th May, Queen Victoria's birthday. Nearby is the Mausoleum of Victoria Mary Louisa (1786–1861), Duchess of Kent, the mother of Queen Victoria. The mausoleum was begun during her lifetime and completed in the year of her death. It was designed by Humbert, with Grüner taking responsibility for the decorative scheme, which included a statue of the Duchess by the

sculptor William Theed. (Photograph of Duchess of Kent's mausoleum on page 3, and of Royal Mausoleum on page 7.)

BUCKINGHAMSHIRE
Chenies
At St Michael's Church is the family mausoleum of the Russells, who were first Earls, then Dukes, of Bedford, and owned the nearby manor house as well as Woburn Abbey. The Bedford Chapel, built by the family in 1556, contains a superb collection of funerary sculpture covering five centuries but can be seen only through a screen.

Fawley
In the churchyard of St Mary's Church are two impressive family mausoleums. The larger is the Freeman mausoleum, which was built in 1750. Its hefty, domed drum is set on an octagonal base, the whole being carried out in pale grey ashlar. The Freemans lived at nearby Fawley Court, which was built for them from 1684. The house was later extended by the Mackenzies, a Scottish banking family, whose mausoleum was erected in the churchyard in 1862. (Photograph of Freeman mausoleum on page 5.)

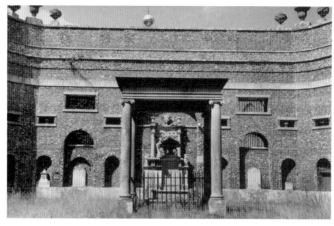

The architect of the weird Dashwood mausoleum at West Wycombe in Buckinghamshire is unknown, although the stonemason John Bastard was paid for his work on the building during 1764–5. The mausoleum was funded by one of Dashwood's Apostles, the group later known as the Hell-Fire Club; given Sir Francis Dashwood's interest in architecture, it seems possible that he at least had a hand in the unique design of his mausoleum.

Hambleden

Two small, stone-built, mid-eighteenth-century mausoleums stand in the churchyard of St Mary's Church in this pretty village. The Kenrick mausoleum, put up by Clayton Kenrick for his father, John, and sister, Elizabeth, has an octagonal dome, while across the churchyard is the Lane family mausoleum, square with a pyramid cap.

West Wycombe

One of the oddest of all British mausoleums, the Dashwood mausoleum

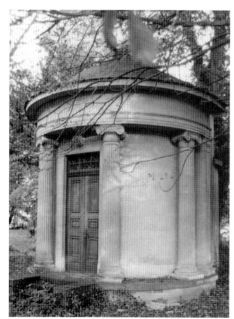

occupies a spectacular site – originally a hillfort – with superb views over West Wycombe Park to the south. West Wycombe House was altered and expanded by Sir Francis Dashwood (1708–81), founder of what later became known as the Hell-Fire Club, who also had a strong interest in architecture. The mausoleum is set beside the church of St Lawrence, whose tower was transformed into an eye-catcher by the addition of a golden ball in 1752, a Christmas tree bauble of unlikely proportions; ten people could be seated within. The roofless, hexagonal rubble-stone (mostly flint) mausoleum was one of the largest in Europe when built around 1765; an urn rests beneath a canopy at its grassy centre, which resembles a setting for some obscure game rather than a conventional mausoleum.

CAMBRIDGESHIRE
Newton

The mausoleum to the south of St Margaret's Church was built in 1922 for Sir Charles Walston of Newton Hall; it was designed by Sir Ambrose Poynter (1867–1923) using a rather dated neo-classical style. Poynter, a member of the Art Workers' Guild, began architectural practice in 1893; he was a cousin of both Stanley Baldwin and Rudyard Kipling.

Waresley

In the midst of estate cottages stands the church of St James, built by William Butterfield in 1855–7; the Duncombe mausoleum, with its unusual almond-shaped

The Walston mausoleum, Newton, Cambridgeshire, was designed by Sir Ambrose Poynter in 1922; the little classical rotunda has an Ionic colonnade topped by a shallow conical roof.

motifs, connects to the north side of the church and was put up soon after the church's completion.

CORNWALL
Madron
The Price mausoleum, built around 1820 in the Greek style, stands in the churchyard of St Madern's Church.

Pentillie Castle
Just inside Cornwall, above the Tamar valley, is the wonderfully chilling tower mausoleum built by Sir James Tillie of Pentillie Castle in 1712. The tower was sited on top of Mount Ararat, just north of the castle, and Sir James was laid to rest there, port in hand, awaiting the Day of Judgement. Those with the courage to peep through the stone grille into the ruined tower may think they see the remains of his body, still waiting.

Treslothan
The Gothic Pendarves mausoleum stands in the churchyard of St John's Church, which was originally the chapel to Pendarves House.

CUMBRIA
Bardsea
The Braddyll mausoleum (NGR: SD 297751) is set high on a hill with vast views over Morecambe Bay to the south-east and Conishead Priory, eventual home of its builder, Colonel T. R. Gale Braddyll, to the north. The architect Philip Wyatt (d.1835) began building the magnificently Gothic Priory (now a Buddhist religious centre) in 1821; he was imprisoned for debt in 1833, and work was finally completed in 1836. A grotto, the mausoleum, several other nearby eye-catchers and a tunnel were erected by the Colonel while the Priory was under construction. The mausoleum, which can just be seen from the road below, is a curious, craggy triangular structure with tiny pyramids capping the corners and niches on each face; weathering has rendered the inscriptions unreadable.

Lowther
The remote Lowther mausoleum, built for William Lowther (1787–1872), Earl of Lonsdale, in 1857, is a handsome Gothic pile, teetering on the edge of a sharp drop to the river Lowther. In the distance are the glowering ruins of Lowther Castle, rebuilt in 1806–11, while just to the north is St Michael's Church. Inside the mausoleum, in a conservatory-like space, is the pale, brooding marble figure of Sir William, staring glumly towards the church; the sculptor (in 1863, well before the Earl's death) was E. B. Stephens. (Photograph on page 40.)

Wreay
The Losh mausoleum (NGR: NY 435489) was built in 1850 by Sara Losh (1785–1853) for her sister, Katherine, who died in 1835. Sara also designed and built the idiosyncratic St Mary's Church in 1840–2; both inside and out, a huge range of naturalistic motifs are used with abandon. The carvings and other decoration were carried out by Sara herself, her cousin and local craftsmen. The church is a tribute to Sara's architectural imagination and the flair of the local labourers; the fact that its unprecedented style and symbolic language were ignored by later architects is a loss to us all. The mausoleum, a monumental construction of irregular stone blocks, is to death as the church is to life; look through its

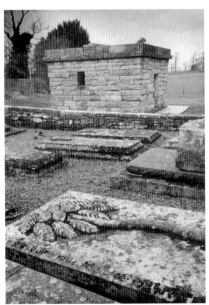

The Losh mausoleum, Wreay, Cumbria, is a massive, squat stone box with barred windows, separated by an enclosure of carved gravestones from Wreay church. The church is one of the most unusual in Britain, its eaves swirling with naturalistic carvings of animals. The mausoleum, built by Sara Losh in 1850, stands near the heavily carved 'runic cross', erected around 1835 in honour of Sara's parents, John and Isabella Losh.

The clean white lines of the Harvey mausoleum, built in 1895 by the firm Harry Hems, make a striking contrast to weather-beaten graves in St Andrew's churchyard, Harberton, Devon. Inside the church, where lavish late-Victorian restoration work is apparent, is a monument – again by Hems – to Robert 'Tito' Harvey, who died in 1895, aged eleven. He also appears in the mausoleum, along with figures of Sir Robert and Lady Harvey.

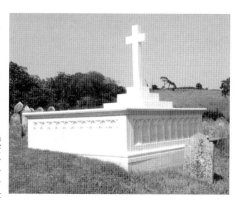

window – if you dare – to be confronted by a cool, white alabaster vision, a statue of Katherine when young. It was sculpted by David Dunbar in 1850 from a sketch made by Sara when the sisters were on holiday in Italy during 1817. It comes as no surprise to find that Sara was eventually buried next to her sister.

DERBYSHIRE
Morley
The Sacheverell-Bateman mausoleum (now in the care of the Mausolea and Monuments Trust) was built in 1897 by G. F. Bodley; it stands in the churchyard of St Matthew's Church, itself a treasure-chest of medieval and later monuments. A stone tithe barn is nearby.

Wingerworth
Attached to the north side of old All Saints' Church is the family mausoleum of the Hunlokes, built in 1783 and very plain; it now acts as a vestry to the new church put up in the 1960s.

DEVON
Bicton
The Rolle mausoleum on the Bicton estate is a perfect little Pugin structure, commissioned by Louisa, Lady Rolle, in 1850 to mark the death of her husband, John, Lord Rolle, in 1842. A. W. N. Pugin used the ruins of a chapel in the medieval Holy Trinity Church as a basis for the mausoleum, creating a superbly ornate interior, which included a tile pavement of mainly blue and yellow Minton encaustics decorated with Rolle initials and emblems, a painted roof, stained glass by Hardman, and elaborate monuments. Though small, it is one of Pugin's most important works.

Harberton
The lightly Gothic Harvey mausoleum in the churchyard of St Andrew's Church is an essay in white marble: not only was it constructed of the material in 1895, but inside it are three recumbent white marble Harveys. The mausoleum was built by the prolific ecclesiastical sculpture firm of Harry Hems of

Exeter, while the figures (by another firm, Toft's) were apparently a tribute to Lady Harvey's Latin-American origins. Dundridge, the Harvey family home, is nearby.

DORSET
Christchurch
The Perkins mausoleum is now but a ruined wall standing in the Priory Gardens, Church Street. The Gothic structure was originally built in 1783 for one Mrs Perkins, who had a mortal fear of being buried alive. She wished her body to be interred above ground in the mausoleum, so that her cries for help could be heard. However, when her husband died in 1803 her body was removed from the mausoleum; the building was then sold and removed to its present site.

Manston
The domed, somewhat overgrown classical mausoleum north of St Nicholas's Church, in the private grounds of Manston House near the river Stour, was built in 1857. It is not only the mausoleum of the Hanham family, who owned the house, but a monument to the British cremation movement. The first occupants of the mausoleum were the deceased wife (d.1876) and mother (d.1877) of Captain Hanham, both of whom had expressed the wish to be cremated. However, cremation was not widely accepted at that time, and their bodies, suitably protected, were stored in the mausoleum while Hanham attempted to gain permission to send them abroad for cremation. This was not forthcoming, and in October 1882 he burnt the bodies in a specially constructed furnace at Manston. Captain Hanham died the following year and was also cremated; the ashes of all three were placed in the mausoleum.

15

Poole

The Leicestershire squire Charles William Packe (1792–1867) inherited Prestwold Hall, near Loughborough, in 1837. He brought in the architect William Burn to remodel the house during 1842–3 but, after quarrelling with his brother, upon whom the estate was entailed, he abandoned the house and bought the Branksome Park estate on the eastern edge of Poole (almost in Bournemouth). In 1852 Burn was called in to build Packe's new home, Branksome Tower. Packe, who was largely responsible for founding the Bournemouth Public Dispensary in 1859, wished to be buried near his new home rather than at the church of St Andrew on the Prestwold Hall estate with other members of the Packe family. In his will dated 1866 Packe left funds for the construction of a mausoleum, the design of which was to be supervised by his wife, Mrs Packe Reading. Charles William Packe died in 1867; his body was temporarily interred at Kensal Green Cemetery in London. Mrs Packe Reading then engaged Burn to design a mausoleum, which was completed in 1869 and stands at the top of Branksome Dene Chine, off Pinewood Road; it is a substantial stone-built chapel floored with black and white marble. After a succession of difficulties involving consecration of the mausoleum and the entailed land on which it stood, Charles

William Packe's remains were finally interred there in May 1871, joining those of his wife, who died the previous year. Branksome Tower eventually became an hotel but was demolished in 1971, and ownership of the mausoleum was transferred to Poole Borough Council. Restoration of the building, which is listed grade II, was completed in 1993.

DURHAM
Gateshead

The Green mausoleum, in the churchyard of old St Mary's Church, is said to have been built by the Northumbrian architect Robert Trollope (d.1686) for his own use. Trollope's style could perhaps be described as bastard baroque, and thus the generous, chunky obelisk finials of the mausoleum (rebuilt in the 1850s for the Green family) could well be his work. He certainly knew how to choose a site for his mausoleum, which has a splendid view of the Tyne and the city across the water.

Rowlands Gill

The chapel on the Gibside estate is also the mausoleum of George Bowes (1701–60), successful businessman and creator of the Gibside landscape. His original intention was to build a mausoleum for his first wife, who died in 1724 after only a few months of marriage, but this wish was never fulfilled

The Green mausoleum, once mouldering away in its Gateshead churchyard overlooking the Tyne, is about to become a near neighbour of the new Sinfonia Centre; in addition, St Mary's Church has taken on a new identity as the Gateshead Quays Visitor Centre. The mausoleum itself dates from the late seventeenth century, but its brickwork was much modified during 1855–60 for the Green family.

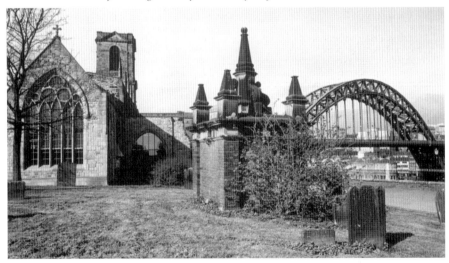

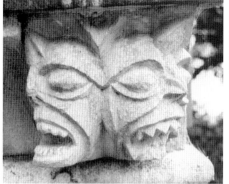

These bug-eyed monsters with their serrated teeth grace the nineteenth-century Iremonger mausoleum at St Peter's, Wherwell, Hampshire. They were originally corbels in the medieval church, which was rebuilt in 1856–8 by the architect Henry Woodyer.

and work only began on the chapel as Bowes's health was failing in 1759. The circular burial vault beneath the chapel measures 10 feet (3 metres) in height and 28 feet (8¹/₂ metres) in diameter. The body of George Bowes was interred in nearby Whickham church until work on the fine stone vault was completed. (Photograph on page 4.)

Staindrop
The village lies in the valley below Raby Castle, which was much altered during the 1840s by the second Duke of Cleveland in conjunction with his architect William Burn. The Vane mausoleum, built in 1850 by Burn for the second Duke, is a little Gothic stone shed, almost hidden by greenery, on the far side of St Mary's churchyard. The church stands on the edge of the Raby estate and has a fine interior with many family monuments.

GLOUCESTERSHIRE
Elmore
Elmore is a tiny hamlet on the banks of the Severn. In the corner of St Mary's churchyard – which has some excellent chest tombs – is the ruined eighteenth-century Guise family mausoleum, once a pyramid-topped arcade guarding the vault.

HAMPSHIRE
Farnborough
One of the most curious mausoleums in Britain is that of Napoleon III, last Emperor of France, his Empress, Eugenie (d.1920), and their son, Louis Napoleon, the Prince Imperial (d.1879). It stands in the grounds of Farnborough Hill, the house (now a school) built around 1862 for the publisher T. G. Longman and bought by the Empress in 1881. She and her architect, Hippolyte Destailleur, built St Michael's Abbey (1876) and the nearby domed mausoleum (1887), the latter in a

flowery French Gothic never taken up by English architects. The mausoleum's vaulted crypt contains three plain tombs.

Hursley
The brick-built Heathcote family mausoleum (1771) is at All Saints' Church, which was rebuilt in 1846–8 for John Keble, leader of the Oxford Movement and vicar of Hursley 1836–66.

Nether Wallop
In St Andrew's churchyard is the mausoleum of the surgeon Francis Douce, who died in 1769 aged eighty-five; it was designed by John Blake of Winchester and built in 1748. Its form – a stone pyramid topped by a flame, signifying eternal life – results from Douce's study of Egyptian burial rituals, combined with the fear that his remains might be disturbed before his expected resurrection. At the centre of the pyramid is a burial chamber in which the body of Douce was deposited, joining that of his wife, who predeceased him. After the second interment the chamber was sealed, as Douce stipulated that he should be the last person buried within.

Old Alresford
The pedimented temple in St Mary's churchyard is the Schwerdt mausoleum; inside is an Italian relief dating from around 1500. Exactly when the mausoleum was built is unclear. It was erected for C. F. G. R. Schwerdt, who apparently died in 1839, but building plans exist dated 1931 and the structure could have been put up during the 1930s using older materials.

Wherwell
The Iremonger mausoleum stands in the churchyard of St Peter and Holy Cross Church; the substantial stone-built structure

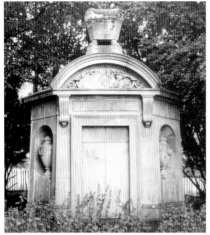

The Lytton mausoleum in Knebworth Park was designed in 1817 by the prolific architect J. B. Papworth, who specialised in the alteration and decoration of country houses. Near the mausoleum is the church of St Mary and St Thomas, where the chapel on the north side of the chancel was rebuilt around 1705 specifically to house the impressive series of Lytton family monuments. Construction of the mausoleum, near the church but not within it, was a response to the movement away from church burial that took hold in the late eighteenth century.

Robert Mylne (1733–1811) for his family in 1800. Mylne, who built himself a house in the village during 1794–7, was buried in the crypt of St Paul's Cathedral, near Sir Christopher Wren, at his own request; he was appointed surveyor of St Paul's in 1766.

has a steeply pitched roof and appears to be late Victorian. There is an ornate opening in the entrance front, above a cusped doorcase.

HERTFORDSHIRE
Ayot St Lawrence

The new St Lawrence's Church was built by Sir Lyonel Lyde in 1778–9, his architect being Nicholas Revett, pioneer of the Greek revival style. The outcome was a very fashionable and truly Greek temple, its façade faced with stucco to act as an eye-catcher (the rear was brick); Sir Lyonel had previously wrecked the village church, which was in the wrong place in relation to his house. Colonnades connect the temple with a pair of pavilions, which act as mausoleums and cover the tombs of Sir Lyonel and his wife.

Great Amwell

In the churchyard on the hill are several large memorials, including the Cathrow mausoleum – a Greek sarcophagus – and the white brick mausoleum built by the architect

Knebworth

The Lytton mausoleum, just east of the church in Knebworth Park, was designed for Mrs Bulwer Lytton in 1817 by the versatile architect and designer J. B. Papworth; the little stone building is crowned by a large sarcophagus. In 1813 Mrs Bulwer Lytton partly rebuilt Knebworth House, which was reconstructed around 1844 by the novelist Edward Bulwer-Lytton (1803–73), who is buried in Westminster Abbey.

KENT
Birchington

The Waterloo Tower in the grounds of Quex Park is a tall, turreted red-brick bell tower topped by an astounding openwork spire in cast iron. Two rooms at the base of the tower form a mausoleum dedicated to Henry Horace Powell Cotton by his son in 1896, but the tower itself was built in 1818–20; the spire is probably contemporary and thus is an unusual early example of cast-iron construction.

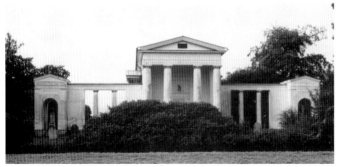

The Lyde mausoleums are the wing pavilions of the new church at Ayot St Lawrence, Hertfordshire. This early Greek revival style church was built in 1778–9 by the architect Nicholas Revett. The body of Sir Lyonel Lyde lies beneath one pavilion, that of his wife beneath the other; apparently their marriage was not altogether happy.

18

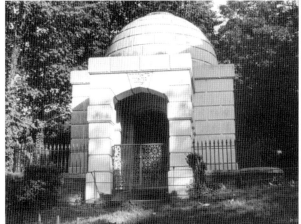

The Montefiore mausoleum, Ramsgate, Kent, was built for the wife of the Jewish philanthropist Sir Moses Montefiore soon after her death in 1862. The design of the mausoleum – a domed, heavily rusticated and stuccoed rectangular structure – was based on the tomb of Rachel, near Bethlehem, which Lady Judith Montefiore had restored.

Boughton Monchelsea

The Walker Head mausoleum stands in the north-east corner of St Peter's churchyard, which has a superb view over the Weald. The domed, stone-built mausoleum was put up around 1838 for the Walker Head family, who lived at Wierton Place.

Chiddingstone

In St Mary's churchyard is a large, pyramid-roofed sandstone mausoleum designed in 1736 by Henry Streatfeild for his family, who lived at High Street House (which was transformed into Chiddingstone Castle, complete with some fine garden buildings, in the early nineteenth century).

Cobham

The magnificent Darnley mausoleum has fallen on sad times, its interior gutted and its approaches neglected. It was built around 1783-4 by James Wyatt for the fourth Earl of Darnley, who inherited Cobham Hall in 1781, but its thirty-two coffin shelves were never occupied. The mausoleum, a classical temple topped by a strange, stark pyramidal roof, was constructed of Portland stone on a square plan with chamfered corners, each of these being capped by a small tomb chest above the entablature. The main room, above the basement coffin chamber, is a circular chapel.

Farningham

In St Peter's and St Paul's churchyard is the mausoleum of Thomas Nash (d.1778), a delicate Portland stone box topped by an obelisk above a dome. Building work on the mausoleum commenced while Nash, uncle of the architect John Nash, was still alive, and was completed after his death.

Ramsgate

The early-nineteenth-century Dunmore (or D'Este) mausoleum, which stands in the churchyard of St Laurence's Church, is a stubby Greek cross in plan; its rather dull sandstone exterior is enlivened by inscribed plaques on three of its four gable ends, revealing the names of those within. It was erected by Augustus Frederick D'Este (1794–1848) as a mausoleum for his mother, Lady Augusta Murray, the morganatic wife of Prince Augustus Frederick, sixth son of George III. Lady Augusta, second daughter of John, Earl of Dunmore, married the Prince in 1793; the remains of their only son are also interred in the mausoleum. Here too are the remains of John Murray (1732–1809), fourth Earl of Dunmore, who became Governor of New York in 1770, his wife, Lady Charlotte (d.1818), and Augusta Emma D'Este (d.1866), only daughter of the Prince and Lady Augusta, and second wife of Thomas Wilde, Baron Truro, Lord Chancellor 1850-2.

Beside the synagogue in Honeysuckle Road is the Montefiore mausoleum, built for Lady Judith Montefiore (d.1862), wife of Sir Moses Montefiore (1784–1885), who financed the synagogue. The interior is top-lit, using coloured glass, and contains the plain marble tombs of Sir Moses and Lady Judith. The mausoleum design was based on the tomb of Rachel, near Bethlehem; the strange stone column at the rear is a reference to the pillar set upon Rachel's grave by Jacob (Genesis 35: 20).

Whitstable

The Ellis mausoleum – a beautifully detailed little classical temple in All Saints' churchyard – was built in 1875 by Charles

Barry junior following the death in 1872 of the wife of Wynne Ellis (1790–1875), art collector and London silk merchant.

LANCASHIRE
Liverpool
In the City of Liverpool Cemetery on Walton Road is the fine grey granite Egyptianate mausoleum built for Alexander McLennan (d.1893) and his wife (d.1896); it stands north-west of the point where the two main paths cross.

Thurnham
The Roman Catholic church of St Thomas and St Elizabeth was built for Elizabeth Dalton of Thurnham Hall in 1847–8. Just north of the church, in the Catholic cemetery, is a spectacularly Egyptianate mausoleum built for the Gillow family, the leading cabinet-making firm from Lancaster, around 1830. The ruddy sandstone mausoleum, whose architect is unknown, was first used in 1836. The Dalton family mausoleum was not at the church but 3 miles (5 km) west across the flatlands south of the Lune estuary, on the coast at Cockersand Abbey. The remains of its thirteenth-century chapter house were converted to a burial chamber for the Daltons in the mid eighteenth century.

LEICESTERSHIRE
Belvoir Castle
The mausoleum stands south of the castle, at the end of a tree-lined avenue. The small, Romanesque structure was built around 1826–8 by Benjamin Dean Wyatt for the fifth Duke of Rutland; soon after its completion, Wyatt turned down the opportunity to design what eventually became Kensal Green Cemetery. He proposed to use the Greek style for the Rutland mausoleum, but the family preferred Norman as this mirrored the origins of the castle. Inside, there is lavish Romanesque stonework theatrically top-lit in purple and yellow.

Buckminster
The Dysart mausoleum, a large Gothic hulk dating from around 1878, stands in St John's churchyard; nice detailing includes iron strapwork on the door, hefty buttresses and a little polychromatic stonework.

LINCOLNSHIRE
Great Limber
The mausoleum built for Sophia Aufrere of Brocklesby Park stands 2 miles (3 km) south of the house in Mausoleum Woods, almost in the village of Great Limber; sited above the park, it has a commanding view over the estate. The circular classical temple was erected in 1792 by C. A. Pelham in memory of his wife, Sophia, who died – aged only thirty-three – in 1786; the architect was James Wyatt. Inside is a statue of Sophia by Joseph Nollekens and the tombs of three other members of the Pelham family. This ravishing mausoleum is one of Wyatt's best works.

LONDON AND MIDDLESEX
Brixton
The monumental mausoleum of Richard Budd (1748–1824) stands at the foot of Brixton Hill, between the Town Hall and the Tate Central Library. It was designed by R. Day in Greek revival style, with three distinct stages topped by a substantial finial of anthemium ornamentation. Budd's youngest son, Henry, who erected the memorial, is also interred within.

Dulwich
The mausoleum at Dulwich Picture Gallery, Gallery Road, SE21, built by Sir John Soane in 1811–14, houses the bodies of the art collector Noel Desenfans (1745–1807), his wife (d.1814) and the artist Francis Bourgeois (1756–1811), landscape painter to George III. Desenfans

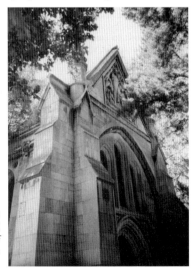

The north gable of the chapel-like Glenesk mausoleum, East Finchley Cemetery, London, with its carving of Christ flanked by angels and soldiers. Inside, the limestone is a rich, deep buff colour; there is a mosaic floor and a colourful reredos, with much stained glass. This fine building was put up in 1899.

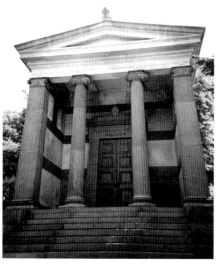

The monumental granite and Portland stone Mond mausoleum, St Pancras and Islington Cemetery, East Finchley, was designed by Darcy Braddell – once a pupil of Ernest George – in the early years of the twentieth century; it was intended as an eye-catcher for the cemetery. Inside are relief plaques of the industrial chemist and art collector Ludwig Mond (1839–1909) and his wife.

had been commissioned to form a national art collection by King Stanislaus of Poland; when Stanislaus abdicated following Poland's partition in 1795, Desenfans was left with the collection. He and his wife shared their London house with Bourgeois, who had been court painter to the Polish king. On the death of Desenfans, Bourgeois inherited the art collection; the will also required that a vault be built for the coffin of Desenfans. Sir John Soane produced a design for a chapel capable of accommodating three coffins, but it was never built. Bourgeois died in 1811, leaving the art collection to Dulwich College and funds to build a picture gallery and a mausoleum for himself and Mr and Mrs Desenfans. Soane was eventually commissioned to build the combined gallery and mausoleum. The gallery is Britain's oldest public picture gallery, and the weirdly gloomy mausoleum – restored with the gallery in 1999–2000 – is an integral part of its structure. The style of the mausoleum combines Greek and Regency, its dome being lit by yellow light; it is at once personal to Soane and perfect in its architectural treatment of death.

East Finchley

The Gothic Glenesk mausoleum on Central Avenue at the East Finchley Cemetery (previously known as St Marylebone Cemetery), East End Road, N2, is the centrepiece of an otherwise completely unremarkable cemetery; it was built in 1899 by Sir Arthur Blomfield. The colourful interior (much of the decoration was by Powell's of Whitefriars) centres on a huge stone sarcophagus, with two smaller tombs by its side; these are for Algernon Borthwick (1830–1908), Lord Glenesk, proprietor of the *Morning Post*, his wife, Alice (d.1898), and son, Oliver (d.1905).

St Pancras and Islington Cemetery lies beside High Road, East Finchley, N2; tucked away on Chapel Hill, at its south-east corner, is the overbearing Mond mausoleum, its design derived from the Hellenistic temple of Nemesis at Rhamnus. Despite its size, locating it is difficult because of the abundance of mature woodland in the cemetery; this makes for a largely undramatic setting, with many modern graves. There are a handful of smaller mausoleums near the south gate, including the Payne mausoleum, built from massive stone blocks.

Forest Gate

The circular, domed Rothschild mausoleum at the Jewish Cemetery within West Ham Cemetery, Cemetery Road, Forest Gate, E7, is a fine building by the architect Sir Matthew Digby Wyatt. It was erected in 1866 by Ferdinand de Rothschild (1839–98) for his wife, Evelina, who died in that year. De Rothschild owned Waddesdon Manor, Buckinghamshire, which was built for him during 1874–89 by Hippolyte Destailleur, the French architect who designed the mausoleum of Napoleon III at Farnborough in 1887.

Golders Green

There are four columbaria (buildings with niches for storing cinerary urns) in the main complex of buildings at Golders Green Crematorium, Hoop Lane, NW11; to the south

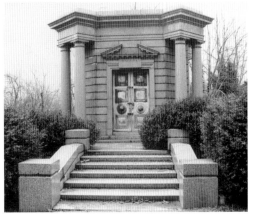

The Dalziel mausoleum in Highgate Eastern Cemetery is constructed from pink granite, its octagonal form being accentuated by the four pairs of Doric columns set on its shorter sides. The bronze doors have lion-head bosses and the interior is lit by a central skylight. Lord Dalziel, who had financial interests in transport, rubber and publishing, introduced Pullman carriages to Britain's railways.

are the Philipson family mausoleum (Sir Edwin Lutyens, 1914) and the Martin Smith mausoleum (1904–5) by Paul Phipps, once an assistant to Lutyens.

Greenwich

The Greenwich Hospital Mausoleum, off Romney Road, SE10, near the National Maritime Museum, was put up in 1750 by Thomas Ripley while he was still working on the Hospital's Queen Mary Court, which he completed the following year. This unassuming brick structure, now restored, formed the entrance to a vault (now bricked up) that extended nearly 30 feet (9 metres) westward beneath the adjoining burial plot. It incorporated a mechanical lift for lowering heavy coffins into the vault; over eighty people, all with some connection to the Hospital, had been interred in the mausoleum by 1842.

Highgate

The outstanding mausoleum in the Western Cemetery, Swains Lane, N6 (open only to guided tours), is that of Julius Beer (1836–80), which was designed by John Oldrid Scott and

based on the original mausoleum at Halicarnassos. Beer, who owned the *Observer*, commissioned the mausoleum in 1876. Others include the Hartley family mausoleum, a huge grey granite Egyptianate building put up in 1860, and the temple mausoleum of Henry Eaton, Lord Cheylesmore, dating from around 1891. Across the road in the Eastern Cemetery there are few memorable tombs apart from the extraordinary Marx edifice, although there is a rather bizarre group of three shiny polished pink granite mausoleums at the entrance, all classical in style; the octagonal one was erected for the financier Davison Dalziel

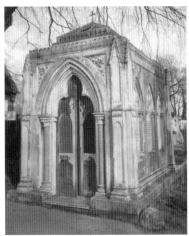

Above: *The late-nineteenth-century Gatti mausoleum, St Mary's Roman Catholic Cemetery, Kensal Green, London, is Gothic with a Byzantine flavour. Its interior is eerily lit by a skylight of mauve and yellow glass.*

Below: *The Molyneux mausoleum, Kensal Green Cemetery, London, is a huge octagonal construction with angel corbels, an abundance of crocketed gables and pinnacles, and a massive bronze door; it was originally topped by a spire. The Gothic pile was built for the otherwise unmemorable Edmund Molyneux (d.1864) in 1866.*

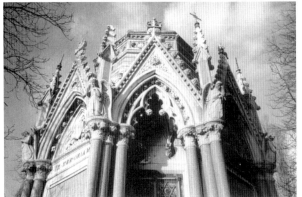

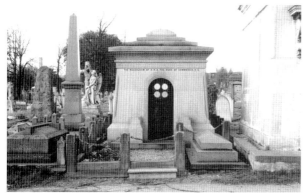

In contrast to the wilful designs of some mausoleums in Kensal Green Cemetery, London, the Duke of Cambridge's Egyptianate mausoleum is very plain. Like his uncle, Prince Augustus Frederick (see Ramsgate, Kent), the Duke made a morganatic marriage. He and his wife, an actress, lie together in the mausoleum.

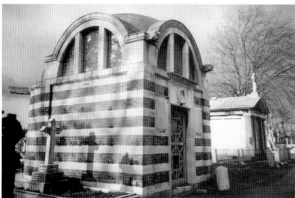

J. D. Campbell's family mausoleum at St Mary's Roman Catholic Cemetery, Kensal Green, London. The strongly polychromatic exterior has survived well, but the interior is in a sorry state, its altar smashed. However, the golden mosaic ceiling is intact, along with its delicately coloured stained glass, out of reach of the vandals.

(1854–1928), Lord Dalziel of Wooler. Highgate, however, is far from the best London cemetery for mausoleum spotting.

Kensal Green

Kensal Green Cemetery, Harrow Road, NW10, was the first of the great nineteenth-century urban cemeteries; it opened in 1833. There are many unusual and architecturally significant tombs, but the major mausoleums are generally sited along Centre Avenue, east of the crossing with Junction Avenue. Amongst them is the pinnacled pink granite Molyneux mausoleum, designed by the architect John Gibson in 1866; close by is Gibson's own mausoleum, a polychromatic tower. He was Grand Superintendent of Works at the cemetery during 1878–82. Just to the west is the idiosyncratic Ducrow

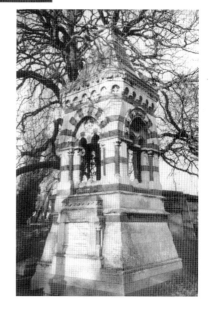

The mausoleum of the architect John Gibson (1817–92) at Kensal Green Cemetery, London, built to his own design. Gibson used a combination of red sandstone and pale limestone, giving a polychromatic appearance to this High Victorian mausoleum.

23

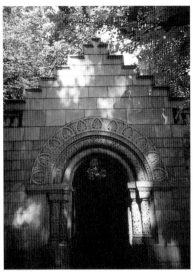

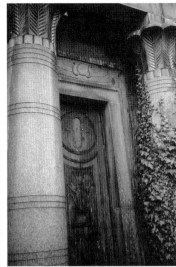

Left:
*Egyptianate
detailing on the
columns and
doorway of the
late-nineteenth-
century Gordon
mausoleum,
Putney Vale
Cemetery,
London. The
bronze door
displays lotus
and cobra motifs.*

Above left: *The crow-stepped gables and ornate Romanesque ornament of the Stearns mausoleum, Nunhead Cemetery, London. The mausoleum was built for Laura Stearns around the time of her death in 1900; it is made from red Doulton terracotta.*

mausoleum, an Egyptianate symbolic mish-mash guarded by sphinxes. Further west on West Centre Avenue is the mausoleum of George William Frederick Charles (1819–1904), second Duke of Cambridge and grandson of George III; it is a plain Egyptianate structure in Peterhead granite. (Photograph of Ducrow mausoleum on page 7.)

The entrance to St Mary's Roman Catholic Cemetery is adjacent to the top gate of Kensal Green Cemetery, on the Harrow Road, NW10. A long avenue leads to the chapel and a group of mausoleums just to the south. These include the Bayona mausoleum, an elegant little Gothic affair that dates from the late nineteenth century, and the Gatti mausoleum, whose occupants include Agostino Gatti (d.1897) and five younger members of the family. Further west is the striking domed polychromatic pile of the Campbell mausoleum; it was built in 1904 by the architect C. H. B. Quennell in Byzantine style. Quennell, who designed several houses in Hampstead Garden Suburb, was also a well-known writer on social history. (Photograph of Bayona mausoleum on page 9.)

Manor Park

The architect of the City of London Cemetery, which opened in 1856 at Aldersbrook Road, Manor Park, E12, was William Haywood (1821–94), who produced a variety of picturesque Gothic structures, one

of which was his own mausoleum. After cremation at Woking his ashes were laid in the mausoleum, which stands on the main avenue north-east of the principal entrance; it has wrought-iron gates and monster gargoyles.

Mortlake

In the Catholic cemetery near St Mary Magdalen Church, North Worple Way, Mortlake, SW14, is the celebrated mausoleum of Sir Richard Francis Burton (1821–90), explorer and scholar, who translated *The Arabian Nights*. It is an 18 feet (5.5 metres) high Bedouin tent in Carrara marble and Forest of Dean stone, designed by his wife, Isabel, Lady Burton (d.1896), who is also interred therein. The mausoleum was built around 1890. The interior shelters their coffins, his being highly enriched, beneath a painted roof representing the heavens; Sir Richard had a horror of darkness. (Photograph on page 8.)

Nunhead

On the hillside path of the wonderfully overgrown Nunhead Cemetery, Linden Grove, SE15, is the Stearns mausoleum, built for Laura Stearns of Twickenham around 1900, although she was buried elsewhere.

Putney Vale

Many of the memorials in Putney Vale Cemetery, Kingston Road, SW15, are rather disappointing in scale, but along the south-

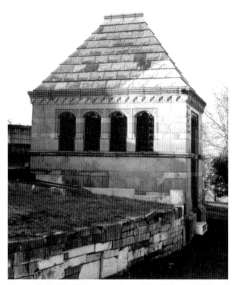 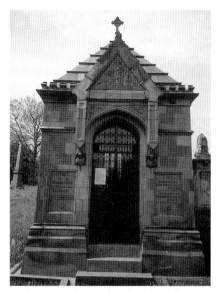

Above left: *The Tate mausoleum, West Norwood Cemetery, London, was built around 1883. The little terracotta shed's interior has a floor of marble and mosaic, while overhead is a golden mosaic ceiling by Powell's of Whitefriars; the frieze around the ceiling is of red and white leaf-patterned glass tiles, and there is also an opus sectile figure of Christ.*

Above right: *The Doulton mausoleum, West Norwood Cemetery, London, was built around 1888 using a combination of Doulton terracotta blocks and miniature bricks. The six green-glazed leaded windows at the sides are protected by wrought-iron grilles of different designs, while the three rear windows were glazed in hand-made Venetian glass. The interior has colourful mosaic work.*

east perimeter path are the massive grey granite mausoleum built for Sir Henry William Gordon (1818–87), brother of General Gordon, and the white marble temple erected for Edwin Tate (d.1928). There is also a late-nineteenth-century mausoleum for the Sainsbury family, in the form of a Doric temple.

Twickenham

The peripatetic Kilmorey mausoleum was originally erected at Brompton Cemetery in 1854, its architect being Henry Edward Kendall (1805–85), son of the architect of the same name who won the competition to design the chapel at Kensal Green Cemetery, although it was never built. Despite its size, the pink and grey granite Kilmorey mausoleum was moved twice before it reached its final resting place near Gordon House (now in educational use), behind a high wall in St Margaret's Road, Twickenham. The second Earl of Kilmorey (d.1880), MP for Newry 1818–26, lived at Gordon House from 1868; his Egyptianate temple was rebuilt at his previous home in 1862, then moved again in 1868. Inside are two coffins, those of the Earl and his mistress, Priscilla Hoste (d.1854).

West Brompton

Brompton Cemetery, Old Brompton Road, SW5, contains many fine tombs, some substantial and highly wrought, but only one which undoubtedly qualifies as a mausoleum. The Courtnoy mausoleum, a daunting Egyptianate mass, lies east of Central Avenue, about halfway between the Great Circle and the north gate; it was built in 1850-2. It is often confused with the Kilmorey mausoleum, of similar bulk and also Egyptianate in style, which was erected at Brompton in 1854 but moved elsewhere in 1862 (see Twickenham).

Westminster

The gardens in Paddington Street, W1, were originally the St Pancras (or St George's) Burial Ground, which opened in 1733; after clearance, one tomb was left because of its fine design. This unprepossessing little classical structure is the mausoleum erected by the Honourable Richard Fitzpatrick for his wife, Susanna (d.1759).

West Norwood

Near the gates of West Norwood Cemetery, off Norwood Road, SE27, is a tall, Portland

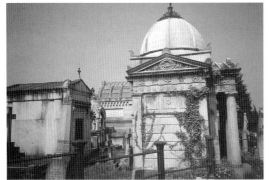

Some of the many mausoleums in the Greek Orthodox Cemetery at West Norwood Cemetery, London. Most prominent here is the temple built for Eustratios Ralli around 1875; at the rear is the J. P. Ralli mausoleum, which contains six shelves bearing velvet-draped coffins.

stone mausoleum with a sweeping curved pyramidal roof and cross-shaped skylights. This elegant structure was built for the surgeon Edmund Distim Maddick (d.1939) in 1931. Just beyond is a small domed mausoleum put up around 1892–3 for Alfred and Elizabeth Longsdon; his name is inscribed above the entrance.

East of the crematorium at the top of the hill is the Tate mausoleum, built around 1883 for the sugar magnate Sir Henry Tate (1819–99) from bright orange-red Doulton terracotta blocks, fitted together in jigsaw-puzzle style; its exterior ornament includes angels and lion heads. The architects were Ernest George and Harold Peto, specialists in the constructional use of terracotta. The mausoleum of Sir Henry Doulton (1820–97), in salmon-pink terracotta made by his own firm, is on the Doulton path just to the south. It was built by George and Peto following Sarah Doulton's death in October 1888. Harold Peto had just completed a country house for the ceramics manufacturer, who then asked Peto to design

a mausoleum similar to Tate's. Peto collaborated with the Italian mosaic artists who had worked on the Tate mausoleum to create another fine decorative interior for the Doulton mausoleum.

The separate Greek Orthodox Cemetery, to the north of the Tate and Doulton mausoleums, has a stunning collection of tombs and mausoleums: almost directly ahead of the gateway is the gigantic J. P. Ralli mausoleum, with a boat-shaped roof on a pink and grey striped granite base. It was designed by G. E. Street soon after 1868 and commemorates John Peter Ralli, who died in 1863 aged one, as well as his father, Peter Ralli (d.1868). Left of the path are the family vault of Ambrose Argenti (1804–71) and then the family vault of T. E. Schilizzi (d.1872) with a standing female figure beneath a baldachin; the large domed temple was built by E. M. Barry for Eustratios Ralli around 1875. There are many other smaller but still notable mausoleums.

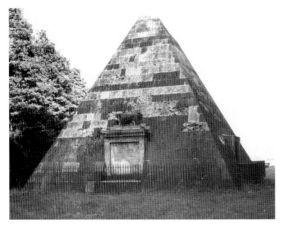

The powerful pyramidal form of the Buckinghamshire mausoleum, Blickling Hall, Norfolk, designed by the architect Joseph Bonomi in 1794 and built during 1796–7. Its base is a 45 foot (14 metre) square.

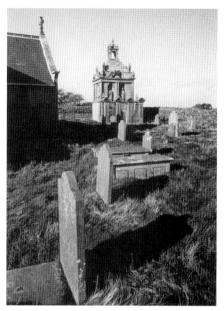

The Hopper mausoleum, at St Andrew's Church on Greymare Hill, near Kiln Pit Hill, Northumberland. There is an expansive view over the county from the 960 feet (293 metres) high churchyard. The designer of this memorable mausoleum, with its oddly carved statues, is unknown.

Wimbledon

In St Mary's churchyard, St Mary's Road, Wimbledon, SW19, north-east of the chancel, is the Portland stone mausoleum of Sir Joseph William Bazalgette (1819-91), the civil engineer responsible for the design of London's sewerage system.

NORFOLK
Blickling Hall

The stark Buckinghamshire pyramid stands about a mile (1.6 km) north-west of Blickling Hall, on the edge of the Great Wood. The mausoleum was built in 1796-7 by Caroline, the second wife of John Hobart (1723-93), second Earl of Buckinghamshire and Viceroy of Ireland. Its domed interior shelters three sarcophagi, for the Earl and his wives.

Ketteringham

The archaeologist Sir John Peter Boileau (1794-1869) bought Ketteringham Hall (now a school) in 1836. Wishing to create a family mausoleum in St Peter's Church, in 1853 he emptied the chancel vaults but was forced to reinstate the coffins and instead built a small brick mausoleum in the churchyard the following year.

Wroxham

The Trafford mausoleum in St Mary's churchyard, built in 1827-8, was an early work of the architect Anthony Salvin; the Trafford family lived at Wroxham Hall, now demolished.

NORTHAMPTONSHIRE
Great Brington

The mausoleum of the Spencers of Althorp is the north chapel of St Mary's Church, which contains monuments to twenty generations of the family. The chapel, built for Sir John Spencer in 1514, is normally locked but the tombs may be seen through the screen. However, the ashes of Diana (1961-97), Princess of Wales, are not at the church but at Althorp, on an island in the ornamental lake known as the Oval. The ashes were placed in an urn mounted on a pedestal, a little way from a small classical memorial pavilion.

NORTHUMBERLAND
Kiln Pit Hill

On Greymare Hill, near the hamlet of Kiln Pit Hill, is the church of St Andrew, and in its isolated churchyard stands the Hopper mausoleum, a jolly confection of statues and obelisks topped by a little lantern. It is said to have been built in 1752 for Humphrey Hopper in memory of his wife, but its rustic style suggests an earlier date.

Kirknewton

In the churchyard of St Gregory's Church is the long stone vault of the Davison mausoleum, built for Alexander Davison (1750-1829), friend of Lord Nelson and owner of nearby Swarland Park.

Seaton Delaval

Seaton Delaval Hall was built by Sir John Vanbrugh for Admiral George Delaval in 1718-29; although fires in 1752 and 1822 destroyed much of its internal fabric, its exterior is still a breathtaking sight. The Delaval mausoleum, now a gaunt, romantic shell, is set in woodland to the east of the house, a little way from other garden buildings. It was built in 1766 by an unknown architect and may be seen from nearby footpaths. (Photograph on front cover.)

NOTTINGHAMSHIRE
Mansfield
The unusual Walker mausoleum (1858) in Mansfield Cemetery is built from massive blocks of stone with minimal decoration.

Milton
Milton is 4 miles (6.5 km) east of Clumber, home of the fourth Duke of Newcastle under Lyme (1785–1851), for whom Sir Robert Smirke built a combined mausoleum and church in 1831–2; it was to contain the tomb of Georgiana, Duchess of Newcastle, who died giving birth to twins in 1822. It was intended to replace an earlier church but has since become redundant and is in the care of the Churches Conservation Trust. The mausoleum, a temple alone in a field, is entered at the east end of the building; although the monument to the Duchess has been removed, the Duke's carved wooden memorial remains.

OXFORDSHIRE
Middleton Stoney
The mausoleum of the Jerseys of Middleton Park was built in 1805 next to All Saints' Church, which at that time stood outside the park. S. S. Teulon created a Norman archway connecting the mausoleum with the chancel in 1858. The gloomy mausoleum contains several memorials, although George Bussy Villiers (1735–1805), fourth Earl of Jersey, for whom it was built, does not appear to have one.

SOMERSET
Bath
The Eyre family chantry and mausoleum at Perrymead Roman Catholic Cemetery (next to the Abbey Cemetery) was built in 1861 by Charles Francis Hansom. It is a substantial Gothic chapel complete with bell tower; the tiled floor of its porch incorporates the Eyre arms.

Chard
The largest monument in Chard Cemetery is the mausoleum of William Moore (d.1901) and his family. Built of white marble and topped by an angel, its interior features a nativity window by A. L. and C. E. Moore; A. L. Moore designed several stained glass windows for London churches around the beginning of the twentieth century.

Claverton
About 4 miles (6.5 km) east of Bath, in St Mary's churchyard at Claverton, is the mausoleum of Ralph Allen (1694–1764); it is a square stone structure with a pyramid roof and was designed by Richard Jones, Allen's clerk of works. Allen, an entrepreneur and philanthropist, created the landscape gardens at his Bath mansion Prior Park, which Jones built and partly designed.

STAFFORDSHIRE
Stone
The architect of Stone's parish church was William Robinson, who produced the design in 1753 while Clerk of the Works at Greenwich Hospital; its construction in 1754–8 was supervised by William Baker, a Cheshire surveyor. In the churchyard stands the classical mausoleum of the Jervis family from nearby Meaford Hall; it was probably also designed by Robinson.

Trentham
It is a shock to the traveller at the end of an everyday bus ride to find, right beside the bus stop, the colossal stone structure that is the Sutherland mausoleum. This hulking neo-classical pile, with its Egyptianate overtones,

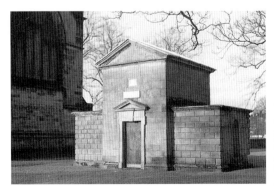

The Jervis family mausoleum at the parish church, Stone, Staffordshire, built in the 1750s and probably designed by William Robinson. One of its occupants is John Jervis (1735–1823), Earl of St Vincent, a native of Stone who became Admiral of the Fleet in 1821.

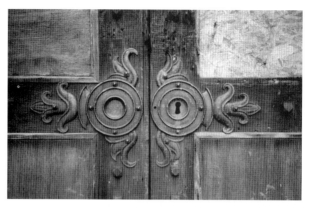

Ironwork detailing on the doors of the Sutherland mausoleum, Trentham, Staffordshire. The mausoleum, which also has ornate wrought-iron entrance gates, was designed by Charles Heathcote Tatham in 1807–8; Tatham was not only an architect but a well-known designer of ornamental metalwork.

reminds the visitor of the lost empire of the Sutherlands: just across the road stood the palatial Trentham Park, rebuilt by the architect Sir Charles Barry in 1833–42 for the second Duke of Sutherland and largely demolished in 1910–12; there are still Italianate remains of some grandeur in what is now Trentham Gardens. The mausoleum was designed by Charles Heathcote Tatham, architect friend of the Duchess of Sutherland, in 1807–8 along with a lodge, bridges and other buildings in Trentham Park. (Photograph on page 6.)

SUFFOLK
Boulge
The church of St Michael stands in the grounds of the now demolished Boulge Hall, home of the Fitzgeralds. Their mausoleum is a low structure in the churchyard, although Edward Fitzgerald (1809–83), translator of *The Rubáiyát of Omar Khayyám*, has a separate grave.

SURREY
Brookwood
The mausoleums at Brookwood Cemetery near Woking, which opened in 1854, include the arcaded Italianate chapel of the Drake family and the domed classical mausoleum erected for George Henry Cadogan (1840–1915), fifth Earl Cadogan, but never used. There are also several mausoleums erected by Parsee families.

Cobham
The ruined Roman Mausoleum at Painshill Park, near Cobham, is one of the many garden buildings (rather than a true mausoleum) in this eighteenth-century landscape.

Egham
The pair of mausoleums in the cemetery at St Jude's Road, Englefield Green, were designed around 1860 by E. B. Lamb for the Fitzroy Somerset family. The polychromatic pair, with their steeply pointed, fishscale-tiled roofs, are like twin gingerbread cottages, typical of Lamb's picturesque style.

SUSSEX, EAST
Brightling
In the churchyard of St Thomas Becket's Church is the monumental, pyramidal mausoleum of John (Mad Jack) Fuller (d.1834), which was built around 1810 and designed by Robert Smirke, who also worked on Fuller's house. Fuller is said to be seated within, wearing a top hat and clutching a bottle of claret.

Brighton
The domed Sassoon mausoleum on the corner of Paston Place is clearly a distant cousin of the Royal Pavilion. It was built in 1892 for the merchant and philanthropist Sir Albert Sassoon (1818–96), who lived in India for many years, and Sir Edward Sassoon (d.1912). It was originally attached to the family home but is now part of the Bombay Arms pub; the Sassoons were buried elsewhere.

Fletching
Edward Gibbon (1737–94), author of *Decline and Fall of the Roman Empire*, is buried in the mausoleum attached to the north transept of the church of St Mary and St Andrew. It was built as a family mausoleum by John Baker Holroyd (1735–1821), first Earl of Sheffield, in the late eighteenth century; Gibbon was a friend of the Sheffields, whose home was nearby Sheffield Place, and the Earl was eventually to edit two of Gibbon's works, both published posthumously.

SUSSEX, WEST

Arundel

The splendid tombs of the Fitzalans (Dukes of Norfolk) of Arundel Castle are visible through an ironwork grille in St Nicholas's Church, which was originally built partly as their mausoleum. As a result of an argument between the church and the Catholic family, a wall was erected in 1879 to separate the Fitzalan Chapel from the rest of the church, but this was taken down in 1969, leaving only the grille. The tombs may be inspected at close quarters from inside the castle grounds.

WILTSHIRE

Bowood

In the grounds of Bowood House is the mausoleum designed by Robert Adam for

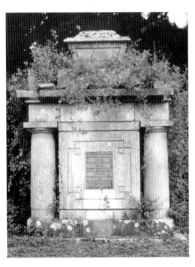

William Petty (1737–1805), second Earl of Shelburne, and completed in 1764; Adam worked on the interiors of the house during 1761–4. Inside the domed, cross-shaped mausoleum is the sarcophagus of the first Earl (d.1761).

Chilton Foliat

In the churchyard of St Mary's Church is the stout stone Pearse mausoleum, now somewhat overgrown; it dates from shortly before 1814.

Trowbridge

Trowbridge General Cemetery, which opened in 1855, has an unusually interesting selection of monuments and mausoleums, including – at its western edge – the pink granite Brown mausoleum, dating from around 1903; its octagonal dome is topped by a tiny ball finial. On the southern perimeter path are the Kingston and Hastings mausoleum, a curious Romanesque design in the form of a long segmental curve above three round-headed arches, and the rather overgrown Rodway mausoleum, put up in 1870. It was designed and built by William Smith of Trowbridge, and its door has superb ironwork.

Westbury

Bratton Road Cemetery, which opened in 1857, has three substantial mausoleums. The most impressive is the octagonal Gothic mausoleum built for John Lewis Phipps (d.1871) of Leighton House; it has a vaulted

Left: The Pearse mausoleum in St Mary's churchyard, Chilton Foliat, Wiltshire. The heavily Greek structure was designed by the London architect and surveyor William Pilkington, who also rebuilt nearby Chilton Lodge for John Pearse in 1800.

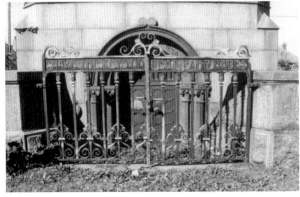

The fine bronze gates and bronze panelled doors of the Brown mausoleum, Trowbridge General Cemetery, Wiltshire, built around 1903. The motto reads, 'I have the keys of Death and Hades'.

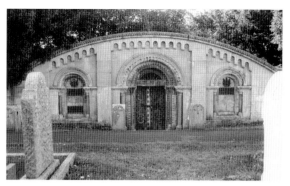

The Kingston and Hastings mausoleum at Trowbridge General Cemetery, Wiltshire, was built by local architect William Smith around the 1870s. The unusual Romanesque design, with its excellent ironwork, was executed for the Reverend Thomas Kingston (d.1867) and the Reverend J. D. Hastings (d.1869), and members of their families.

interior above armorial floor tiles. Near it is the smaller, hexagonal Ludlow mausoleum, built between 1886 and 1900 for Henry Charles Lopes (1828–99), created first Baron Ludlow in 1897. Finally, on the main avenue is the Romanesque chapel known as the Lopes mausoleum, built around 1910.

WORCESTERSHIRE
Ombersley

The Sandys mausoleum, near St Andrew's Church, was originally part of the old church;

new crenellated end walls were added around 1830.

YORKSHIRE, EAST
Halsham

On the northern fringe of the village, at the end of a tree-lined walk opposite the church, is the Constable mausoleum, an elegant round stone temple. It was built in 1792–1802 by Edward Constable, whose family had already left Halsham for Burton Constable Hall, and its architect was Thomas Atkinson; it was his

Right: In the foreground is the tall Gothic Phipps mausoleum, built around 1871 at Bratton Road Cemetery, Westbury, Wiltshire. Close by stands the delicate, hexagonal Ludlow mausoleum, which dates from the late nineteenth century; it is built from rubble-stone.

Below: This Romanesque chapel is the Lopes mausoleum in Bratton Road Cemetery, Westbury, Wiltshire. It was built around 1910 for George Lopes, Baron Ludlow, and his wife, Georgina (d.1912).

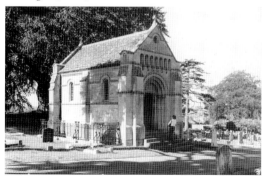

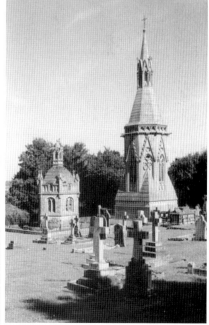

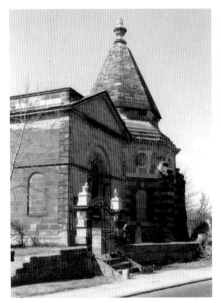

Entrance to the Turner mausoleum at Kirkleatham, North Yorkshire, is via an unexpected doorway in the north side of the chancel of St Cuthbert's Church. The mausoleum's interior is plain (probably a result of its 1839 restoration) and rather dreary, with niches and a central tomb chest, and does not prepare the visitor for the shock of seeing its exterior. The mausoleum's rusticated octagon easily overpowers the more polite architecture of John Carr's rebuilt church.

House (now demolished), the largest of the merchants' houses in Welton, then built the grey brick Welton Manor around 1820.

YORKSHIRE, NORTH

Castle Howard

The grandest of all English mausoleums lies almost a mile (1.6 km) east of Castle Howard and is visible from a footpath running through the grounds. Sir John Vanbrugh, who had seen for himself the immense mausoleums of Mughal India, discussed the construction of a mausoleum with Charles Howard (1669–1738), third Earl of Carlisle, during the early 1720s. After Vanbrugh's death in 1726, Nicholas Hawksmoor took up the idea and produced an initial design by 1728. The foundations were laid in April 1729, but the mausoleum was not completed until 1745, whereupon the Earl's remains were removed to the mausoleum from the local parish church. (Photograph on page 5.)

final building, finished four years after his death. Inside the mausoleum, which is lit by coloured glass, is a frieze of seventy-two painted shields; the Constable remains were transferred from All Saints' to the mausoleum after its completion.

Welton

The circular, domed Raikes mausoleum lies at the wooded head of Welton Dale, not far from the road leading north out of the village, which became popular with Hull merchants in the eighteenth and nineteenth centuries. The mausoleum was built in 1818 for Sir Robert Raikes, a Hull banker who first rebuilt Welton

Kirkleatham

The craggy, octagonal Turner mausoleum dominates St Cuthbert's Church, its pyramidal stone roof reaching well above the eighteenth-century church to which it is attached. It was built in 1740 for the Turners of Kirkleatham Hall (a Jacobean mansion

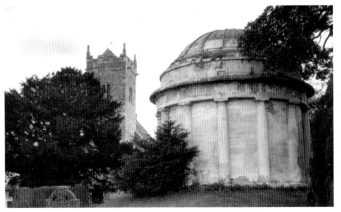

The Thompson mausoleum, Little Ouseburn, North Yorkshire, is a fine example of Palladian style, with its dome and thirteen attached Tuscan columns. It dates from the mid eighteenth century but the architect is unknown.

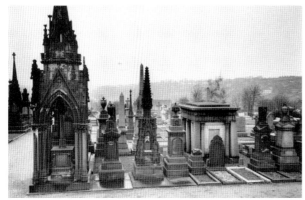

demolished in the 1950s) in memory of Marwood William Turner (d.1739), 'the best of sons' according to the inscription; the architect was James Gibbs. The mausoleum, which was restored in 1839, is entered via a doorway from the chancel.

Little Ouseburn

In the lush graveyard of Holy Trinity Church, almost obscured by trees, is the Thompson mausoleum, built around 1742 by Henry Thompson (d.1760) of nearby Kirby Hall (demolished 1920). Both Hall and mausoleum were evidence of Thompson's enthusiasm for the Palladian style and his friendship with Lord Burlington.

YORKSHIRE, SOUTH
Wentworth

The vast Palladian mansion of Wentworth Woodhouse was completed around 1770 by Charles Watson-Wentworth (1730–82), second Marquis of Rockingham. He also added at least one tremendous folly to an estate strewn with them, although his mausoleum, near Nether Haugh (NGR: SK 414971), was built for Rockingham's heir, Charles, fourth Earl Fitzwilliam. The three-tiered tower with its four outlying obelisks was built by John Carr in 1785–91; however, the mausoleum was never used – Rockingham's body was interred at York Minster. (Photograph on page 1.)

The Holden family mausoleum, on the main promenade of Undercliffe Cemetery, Bradford, West Yorkshire. The little Renaissance pavilion, which has good relief carving, was built for John Holden (d.1849); beyond it is the Behrens mausoleum. Although the cemetery's buildings were demolished in the 1980s, most of the monuments still remain in reasonable condition.

YORKSHIRE, WEST
Bradford

The first impression of the Undercliffe Cemetery, apart from the expansive views over Bradford, is of tremendous verticality, with memorials crushed together and reaching heavenwards like a weird stone forest. One of the tallest is the Albert-Memorial-like Anderton family mausoleum, near the meeting of the main promenade and the curving path from the entrance. Nearby is

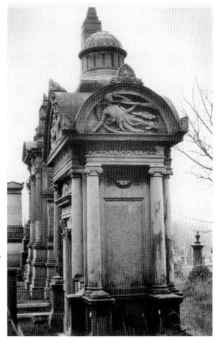

the Egyptianate Illingworth mausoleum, guarded by two sphinxes; it is sited in an enclave of large monuments below the main promenade, which has a superb display of memorials to the wool merchants of Bradford. These include the Behrens and Holden mausoleums, which are separated by an Egyptianate pinnacle. (Photograph of Illingworth mausoleum on page 6.)

Saltaire
The textile manufacturer and philanthropist Sir Titus Salt (1803–76) began to create the model township of Saltaire, centred on his new mill, around 1851, and built its Congregational Church in 1858–9. It was designed by the architects Lockwood and Mawson, who were also responsible for the housing and the architectural styling of the mill. Sir Titus was buried in the domed Salt family mausoleum, which was added to the church by Lockwood and Mawson in 1861. The mausoleum, which has a floor of patterned Minton tiles, is entered from the south aisle of the church.

SCOTLAND
ARGYLL AND BUTE
Gruline, Isle of Mull
In contrast to its romantic leafy setting on the Gruline estate (NGR: NM 549398) in north Mull, the mausoleum erected around 1825 for Major General Lachlan Macquarie (1762–1824) and his family is a dour, windowless stone box. Macquarie was the nephew of clan chieftain Murdoch MacLean of Lochbuie in

south Mull and eventually made his home on the island. He was Governor of New South Wales in 1810–21 and became known as 'The Father of Australia' because he saw the colony as a growing community rather than simply a penal settlement.

Kilmun
The mausoleum of the Dukes and Duchesses of Argyll, built in 1795–6 by James Lowrie, now stands in the lee of the new parish church erected in 1841; the mausoleum's metal dome was an addition of 1891–3. North of the church is the red sandstone Douglas of Glenfinnart mausoleum, put up in 1888.

Lochbuie, Isle of Mull
St Kenneth's Chapel, which dates from around 1500, was rebuilt in 1864 as the mausoleum of the MacLeans of Lochbuie; it stands a mile (1.6 km) south-east of Lochbuie House (NGR: NM 626236). The path around the loch shore eventually brings the visitor to this remote little stone building; the ironwork gate swings open, revealing darkness within and sudden, breathtaking colours above. Magic? No, just part of the 1974 restoration, which included the insertion of star-shaped coloured glass plates into the roof. After the gloom dissipates, a Gothic revival screen can be seen at the east end of the chapel. Another, smaller, mausoleum, just north-west of Lochbuie House, was built in 1777 for the MacLeans.

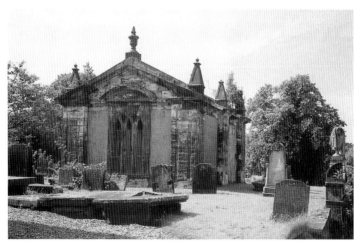

The Bute mausoleum in High Kirk burial ground, high above the town of Rothesay; there is a wonderful view north-east across the Firth of Clyde. The mausoleum, which was built in the eighteenth century, is a stylistic mixture of classical, Gothic and Baroque elements.

34

Rothesay

At the rear of the High Kirk in Rothesay's High Street is the mausoleum built for the Butes of nearby Mount Stuart during the eighteenth century; it is a stylistic mixture in red sandstone.

DUMFRIES AND GALLOWAY

Bentpath

The domed, classical Johnstone family mausoleum in the graveyard of Westerkirk parish church was built by Robert Adam in 1790 for Sir James Johnstone; it was the second mausoleum that Adam had built for the family. The first was designed about a year earlier for John Johnstone, while Adam was carrying out alterations to his home, Alva House; it stands in Alva churchyard, Clackmannanshire.

Closeburn

In the parish churchyard at the planned village of Closeburn is the classical mausoleum built in 1742 for Thomas Kirkpatrick; inside is a skull and crossbones frieze.

Dumfries

The very white domed octagon of the Burns mausoleum stands in a corner of the graveyard at St Michael's and South Church, St Michael Street (to the south of the town centre). It was built by the London architect T. F. Hunt in 1815–16 following a national appeal instigated by Dorothy and William Wordsworth, who had difficulty in finding the grave of the poet Robert Burns (1759–96) when they visited Dumfries in 1803.

Kelton

In woodland just north of the church is the impressively large mausoleum built in 1821 for the businessman and landowner Sir William Douglas (1745–1809) of nearby Gelston Castle (now derelict); its mighty battered walls and double pagoda roof combine Egyptian, Greek and even Japanese styles. The architect may have been Sir William's nephew William Douglas and his companion on the grand tour, the landscape painter Hugh 'Grecian' Williams, or possibly the Dumfries architect Walter Newall. Note the Douglas crest above the doorway; its supporters wear bowler hats.

Kirkland

The village, on the A702 north-west of Dumfries, is dominated by Glencairn parish church; in its churchyard is the early-nineteenth-century Gillespie mausoleum, a petite classical temple topped by an urn upon a dome.

EAST LOTHIAN

Aberlady

The Wemyss mausoleum lies in the grounds of Gosford House, on the shore of the Firth of Forth. The architect of the overbearing classical pyramid is unknown, but it may perhaps have been Robert Adam for it was he who built Gosford House for the seventh Earl of Wemyss in the 1790s.

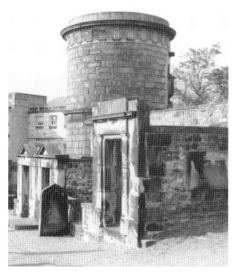

The severe classical drum of the mausoleum built for David Hume (1711–76) in 1778 by Robert Adam at Old Calton Burying Ground, Edinburgh.

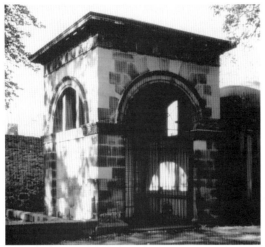

The Adam mausoleum (left) at Greyfriars Churchyard, Edinburgh. The architects John and Robert Adam designed the perfectly classical mausoleum of their father, William Adam (1689–1748), in 1753. Beside it is the mausoleum of William Robertson (d.1793).

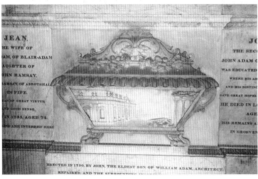

Left: Part of an interior panel in the Adam mausoleum. The tomb chest depicts Hopetoun House, West Lothian, which William Adam enlarged for the Earls of Hopetoun during 1723–48, the work being completed after William's death by his sons.

EDINBURGH
Edinburgh

The mausoleum erected by Robert Adam in 1778 for the philosopher David Hume (1711–76) at Old Calton Burying Ground is a stern, classical stone drum.

Greyfriars Churchyard, Candlemaker Row, is a pleasantly green space, although the Covenanters' Prison (sometimes closed) is a creepy, gloomy passageway that harbours the early-eighteenth-century Adam Brown mausoleum. Beside the south wall of the churchyard is the large, domed Mackenzie mausoleum, erected around 1685–91 and the first conventional mausoleum to be built at Greyfriars. Close by is the fine Little tomb,

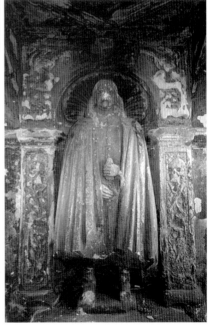

Right: The disturbing figure of John Bayne (d.1681) regards visitors from beneath the heavy canopy of his mausoleum, which stands within an enclosure built in 1684-5 at Greyfriars Churchyard, Edinburgh.

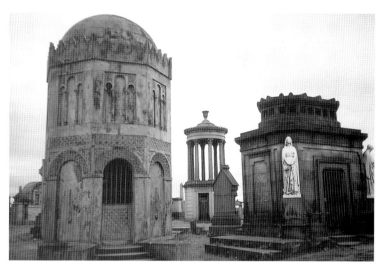

monumental enough to be defined as a mausoleum but lacking the conclusive element of entrance into a building; it is a reclining figure beneath a canopy inside a railed enclosure. Near the Covenanters' Prison are two mausoleums, the larger being that of the architect William Adam; its neighbour is the Robertson mausoleum. At the far northern end of the churchyard are the splendidly eerie

Bayne enclosure and mausoleum; nearby is a dull little stone shed of a mausoleum, built for the Trotters in 1709–10 by Robert Mylne and his son William. Finally, on the east side near the entrance, completing an entire wall of monuments, is the mausoleum put up for John Law (d.1712) and his wife (d.1703), which was restored in 1803. Altogether the churchyard has a strange and wonderful collection of tombs, but its atmosphere is less inspiring than that of a single, solitary mausoleum in the countryside. (Photograph of Mackenzie mausoleum on page 4.)

GLASGOW
Glasgow

The Eastern Necropolis, which overlooks the city from its site above the cathedral on Wishart Street, opened in 1833; the main entrance is through the gateway on Cathedral Square. The most significant mausoleums and monuments are in the oldest part of the cemetery, which was extended eastward in 1854 and again following 1894. On the broad flat hilltop, amongst many other memorials, is the Houldsworth mausoleum, built in 1854 by John Thomas and easily identified by the sculpted figures of Hope and Charity at its entrance. One of the largest mausoleums in

The Monteath mausoleum, built in 1842 at the Glasgow Necropolis. The rich Romanesque stonework detailing by David Cousin is unusual in this cemetery, where classical styles predominate.

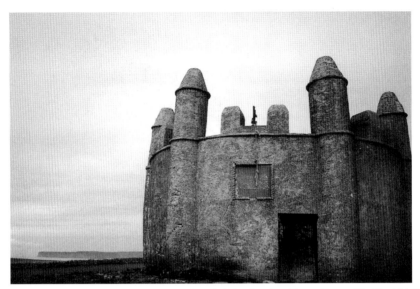

Harold's Tower, the Sinclair mausoleum, on the Hill of Clairdon above Thurso; Dunnet Head is visible in the far distance. In addition to being a mausoleum, the tower commemorates the Norse Earl Harold, who was killed in the battle of Clairdon in 1195 and buried nearby.

the Necropolis is sited where the land drops away to the west: the Monteath mausoleum is a circular Romanesque chapel built in 1842 by David Cousin for Archibald Douglas Monteath. To the south is the ornate Aikens mausoleum, designed around 1875 by James Hamilton II.

HIGHLAND
Duthil
The Seafield family mausoleum, east of the parish church in the little hamlet of Duthil, was built in 1837 by William Henry Playfair.

Harris, Isle of Rum
The Bullough mausoleum, on a clifftop near Harris on the island of Rum, was put up by Sir George Bullough of Kinloch Castle (itself built for the Lancashire industrialist in 1897) in the early twentieth century. The original family vault, just to the north-west, was partially demolished by the family after being likened to a men's lavatory.

Thurso
Harold's Tower, the mausoleum of the Sinclairs of Ulbster, stands high on a hill above Thurso, a tiny castle visible for miles around. It was built in 1780–90 by Sir John Sinclair to supersede the family vault at Ulbster.

Ulbster
In the centre of Ulbster burial ground is the Sinclair mausoleum, a square building with an ogee roof (which hides complex woodwork), erected in 1700 and restored in 1995.

SCOTTISH BORDERS
Ancrum
The Monteath mausoleum lies just west of the A68, a couple of miles (3 km) north of Ancrum (NGR: NT 613268). The site is stunning, with panoramic views of the hills taking in the Waterloo monument on Penniel Heugh to the east. All is wildly romantic, as is the mausoleum itself, a starry, domed temple guarded by a pair of lions, who seemingly take it in turn to snooze. It was built in 1864 for General Sir Thomas Monteath Douglas (1787–1868), whose early army career was in the Bengal Infantry; he took the additional surname of Douglas in 1851.

SOUTH LANARKSHIRE
Hamilton
The colossal mausoleum commissioned by Alexander Hamilton Douglas (1767–1852), tenth Duke of Hamilton, was begun in 1840 by

38

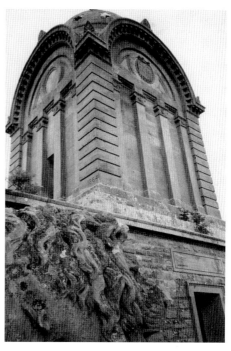

A lion guards the base of the Monteath mausoleum near Ancrum in the Scottish Borders. The mausoleum is a domed, Byzantine temple resting on a vault; the interior is lit by star-shaped glass skylights. It was built in 1864 for Sir Thomas Monteath Douglas of Stonebyres House, Lesmahagow, South Lanarkshire, by the architects Peddie and Kinnear.

the leading Glasgow architect David Hamilton, who also rebuilt the north front of Hamilton Palace for the Duke during the 1820s. The mausoleum was eventually completed by David Bryce to a different design and is basically a drum upon a square, arcaded base. Its huge size and weight caused it to sink 24 feet (7 metres) in the century following its construction. Inside is a chapel guarded by stone lions, with an Egyptianate sarcophagus; the chapel has a fifteen-second echo. The tenth Duke claimed to be the true heir to the Scottish throne.

WALES
CARDIFF
Roath

In 1800 the first Marquis of Bute added a family mausoleum to the church of St Margaret of Antioch, Waterloo Road. However, the church was rebuilt in 1869–70 for the third Marquis of Bute (1847–1900) by the leading church architect John Prichard, and the mausoleum itself was rebuilt by Prichard in 1881–6. The highly polychromatic interior of the church is complemented by the lavish carving of the mausoleum. In the mausoleum, which is separated from the body of the church by an arcade, are unnerving rows of perfectly smooth granite tomb chests.

GWYNEDD
Penygroes

Construction of the massive, circular Newborough mausoleum in Glynllifon Park ceased in the 1830s; Glynllifon was the home of the Lords Newborough. The mausoleum was neither completed nor used; inside are a staircase and many empty rooms.

Further reading

Brooks, Chris. *Mortal Remains*. Wheaton, 1989.

Colvin, H. *Architecture and the After-life*. Yale University Press, 1991.

Craig, Maurice, and Craig, Michael. *Mausolea Hibernica*. Lilliput Press, 1999.

Craske, Matthew. 'Entombed Like an Egyptian', in *Church Monuments*, 15 (2000), pages 71–88. (The Douce mausoleum at Nether Wallop, Hampshire.)

Curl, James Stevens. *The Victorian Celebration of Death*. Sutton Publishing, 2000.

Curl, James Stevens. *A Celebration of Death*. Batsford, 1993.

Hill, Rosemary. 'Romantic Affinities', in *Crafts*, 166 (2000), pages 34–9. (Wreay church and mausoleum.)

Jupp, Peter C., and Gittings, Clare (editors). *Death in England: an Illustrated History*. Manchester University Press, 1999.

Sheridan, Alison (editor). *Heaven and Hell and Other Worlds of the Dead*. National Museums of Scotland, 2000.

Smith, Charles Saumarez. *The Building of Castle Howard*. Pimlico, 1997.

Williams, Robert. 'A Factor in His Success', in the *Times Literary Supplement*, 3rd September 1999, pages 13–14. (Vanbrugh and Mughal mausoleums.)

The Mausolea and Monuments Trust is a registered charity founded in 1997; it is responsible for the upkeep of several mausoleums and produces a regular newsletter. The Trust may be contacted at 24 Hanbury Street, Spitalfields, London SE1 9QR.

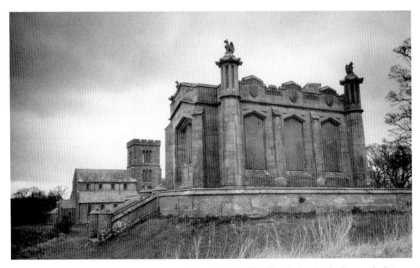

The Lowther mausoleum, Lowther, Cumbria, with St Michael's Church in the background. Between the mausoleum and Lowther Castle to the south stood old Lowther village, pulled down in 1680 by Sir John Lowther to enhance the view of the church. The sandstone and granite mausoleum was erected in 1857, a year after the church was partly rebuilt.